Raw Food Diet Cookbook

By

Cheryl Green

Table of Contents

Chapter 1: Introduction

    What is the Raw Food Diet?

    What are its benefits?

    What are the drawbacks?

    What foods are included?

Chapter 2: Breakfast Recipes

    Raw Chocolate Breakfast Smoothie

    Mango Green Smoothie With Honey

    Banana Pancakes

    Healthy Chocolate Frappuccino

    Strawberry and Flax Breakfast Smoothie

Breakfast Fruit Pizza

Quick and Easy Granola Bars

Blueberry and Banana Breakfast Parfaits

Cinnamon Rolls

Coconut and Pumpkin Spice Energy Bars

Chapter 3: Main Meal and Side Dish Recipes

Chinese Hot and Sour Cole Slaw

Vegan Cream of Mushroom Soup

Ranch Dressing (For Salads, Sandwiches, Etc.)

Carrot Sushi Rolls

Spinach Burgers For the Dehydrator

Raw Food Sandwich Bread

Veggie Sandwich on Onion Bread

Raw Taco Meat Wraps

Raw Gazpacho

Moroccan Salad

Veggie Pasta Marinara

Cauliflower Rice Pilaf

Zucchini Noodles With "Bolognese" Sauce

"Fish" Sticks with Tartar Sauce

Raw Pad Thai

Vegetable Spring Rolls With Spicy Curry Dipping Sauce

Curry Zoodles (Zucchini Noodles)

Egg-Free Egg Salad

Raw Mushroom Burgers With Avocado Mayonnaise

Raw Caesar Salad

Chapter 4: Snack and Dessert Recipes

    Fresh and Easy Guacamole

    Crunchy Coconut Macaroons

    No Bake Strawberry "Cheesecake"

    No Bake Brownies

    Raw Salsa With Raw Corn Tortilla Chips

    Raw Oatmeal Raisin Cookies

    Raw Pumpkin Pie

    Strawberry Ice Cream

    Dark Chocolate Milkshake

    Bean-Free Hummus

Chapter 1: Introduction

What is the Raw Food Diet?

Like the name suggests, the Raw Food Diet is a diet that consists of eating food that is completely raw, unprocessed, and mostly whole plant-based. However, it is acceptable to eat foods that are minimally-cooked, which is around 104 to 118 degrees Fahrenheit. It is also possible to eat raw meat and raw animal products, but most of the people who use this diet are vegans.

What are its benefits?

Studies suggest that being on the Raw Food Diet leads to an increase in energy levels, clearer skin, loss of weight, improved digestion, and reduced risk of diseases. This diet is low in both sodium and sugar, but high in potassium, magnesium, folate, fiber, and Vitamin A, among other things. As a result, you'll find that you are at less risk of getting diseases like diabetes, cancer, and heart-related diseases. You also will yield better blood test results.

What are the drawbacks?

There are nutritional deficiencies that include vitamin B12, iron, zinc and omega-3 fatty acids, which put you at a higher risk for heart disease. However, this can be countered by taking multivitamins and supplements.

Another drawback, as with any diet, is that you may suffer from symptoms of withdrawal, including nausea, cravings, mild headaches, and digestion problems (from the sudden change in diet), which can last for several days but could eventually subside. Therefore if you're going to try this diet, it's a good idea to ease into slowly and make sure to get the approval of a medical professional before starting this diet.

Also note that this diet has not been proven to be safe for women who are pregnant, mothers who are nursing, children, and those with certain medical conditions or are taking certain medications. Therefore, again, you should consult with a doctor before taking on this diet.

What foods are included?

Here are the foods allowed for the Raw Food Diet, separated into categories.

Fruits, such as:

- apples
- oranges
- lemons
- limes
- blueberries
- strawberries
- raspberries
- grapes
- bananas
- avocados
- mangos

- dates

- raisins

Vegetables, such as:

- bell peppers

- kale

- lettuce

- onion

- spinach

- tomatoes

- zucchini

- celery

- alfalfa sprouts

- peas

Dried, raw nuts and seeds, such as:

- sunflower seeds
- almonds
- cashews
- macadamia nuts
- pine nuts
- flax seeds
- chia seeds
- hemp seeds

Grains, such as or coming from products like:

- cereal
- bread
- granola
- millet
- buckwheat
- quinoa
- oats

Oils, such as:

- raw, virgin coconut oil
- cold-pressed, extra-virgin olive oil

Animal products, such as:

- raw eggs*

- non-pasteurized, non-homogenized milk*

- non-pasteurized, non-homogenized yogurt

- non-pasteurized, non-homogenized cheese

- fish*

- beef*

* Note that consuming these might increase the risk of foodborne illnesses in your body

Miscellaneous other foods, including:

- garlic

- ginger

- beans

- freshly-made fruit and/or vegetable juice

- legumes

- purified water

- seaweed

Chapter 2: Breakfast Recipes

Raw Chocolate Breakfast Smoothie

Preparation Time: 5 minutes

Cooking Time: 0 minutes

Total Time: 5 minutes

Servings: 2

Ingredients:

- 2 bananas

- 1 tablespoon hemp seed

- 1 cup frozen blueberries

- 1/2 cup of liquid stevia

- pure water

- 2 teaspoons raw chocolate

- 1/2 teaspoon cinnamon powder

- 1 pinch cayenne pepper

Preparation:

1) Add all of the ingredients to a high-speed blender, putting enough water to cover all of the ingredients.

2) Blend well.

3) Test. If it's too thick for your tastes, add a little more water at a time until your desired consistency.

Mango Green Smoothie With Honey

Preparation Time: 5 minutes

Cooking Time: 0 minutes

Total Time: 5 minutes

Servings: 1

Ingredients:

- 2 bananas, peeled and cut into slices
- 1 large mango, peeled and cut into cubes
- 1 1/2 cups orange juice
- 1 large handful of fresh spinach, chopped up
- 1 generous-sized tablespoon honey

- 3 – 4 ice cubes

Preparation:

1) Blend all of the ingredients in a high powered blender. The number of ice cubes depends on your desired consistency. More ice cubes will make a creamier smoothie.

Banana Pancakes

Preparation Time: 10 minutes

Dehydration Time: 5 hours

Total Time: 5 hours and 10 minutes

Servings: 4 – 5 pancakes

Ingredients:

- 1 large banana

- 1/4 cup raw buckwheat flour

- 2 tablespoons flax meal

- 1 teaspoon cinnamon

- 1/4 cup almond milk

Preparation:

1) Using a food processor or blender, blend all of the ingredients together.

2) Line a dehydrator tray with Teflex.

3) Pour the batter in 1/4 cup spoonfuls onto the prepared tray.

4) Dehydrate them for about 2.5 hours at 115 degrees Fahrenheit.

5) Flip them over and dehydrate for another 2.5 hours at 115 degrees.

Note: Make sure to check often during the dehydration process so that they don't become too hard.

Healthy Chocolate Frappuccino

Preparation Time: 5 minutes

Cooking Time: 0 minutes

Total Time: 5 minutes

Servings: 1

Ingredients:

- 1 banana, frozen and cut into chunks
- 3/4 cup almond milk or milk of your choice
- 1 teaspoon of instant coffee granules or cold brew
- 1 tablespoon raw cacao powder
- 2 – 3 teaspoons maple sweetener or other sweetener of choice

Preparation:

1) Blend everything together using a blender.

Strawberry and Flax Breakfast Smoothie

Preparation Time: 5 minutes

Cooking Time: 0 minutes

Total Time: 5 minutes

Servings: 1 – 2

Ingredients:

- 2 bananas, frozen and then sliced
- 1 cup strawberries, frozen
- 4 tablespoons flax seeds, ground
- 1 cup almond milk
- chopped almonds for an optional garnish

Preparation:

1) Put all of the ingredients into a high-powered blender and blend until smooth using the "puree" button.

2) Garnish with the chopped almonds before serving, if using.

Breakfast Fruit Pizza

Preparation Time: 1 hour

Cooking Time: 0 minutes

Total Time: 1 hour

Servings: 1 pizza

Ingredients:

For the "Crust":

- 2 cups almonds, walnuts, or a mixture of the two

- 8 – 12 Medjool dates, pitted

For the "Sauce":

- 1 1/2 cups cashews

- 1/2 cup water

- 3 tablespoons coconut oil

- 2 tablespoons maple syrup

- 1 tablespoon vanilla extract (alcohol-free, if desired)

For the Toppings:

- assorted fruits of your choice, prepared as follows:

    fruit like kiwi, peeled and cut into thin slices

    fruit like strawberries, cut into thin slices

    round berries, whole or cut up

bananas, sliced into thin slices

other fruit, cut into your preference to look like pizza toppings

Preparation:

For the "Sauce":

1) Blend all of the "sauce" ingredients in a food processor until you get a smooth texture.

2) Transfer it to a bowl. Place the bowl in the fridge for 45 minutes to allow the "sauce" to harden.

For the "Crust":

1) Meanwhile, line the bottom of a tart, cake, or pie pan with parchment paper.

2) Pulse the almonds and/or walnuts using a food processor, until you get a meal that is coarse in texture.

3) With the food processor running, add the Medjool dates one at a time until you form a crust. The amount of dates depends on when you can pick up the dough, and it sticks together between your fingers.

4) Then transfer the dough to the prepared pan and, using your hands, press the dough into the bottom of the pan (only) to form a pizza "crust". Make sure to press it evenly across the bottom of the pan.

5) Place another sheet of parchment paper on top of the dough, and put in the fridge until set, about 20 minutes.

To Assemble:

1) Spread out the "sauce" first.

2) Then lay out the fruit like pizza toppings.

3) Cut into slices and serve.

Quick and Easy Granola Bars

Preparation Time: 5 minutes

Setting Time: 30 minutes

Total Time: 35 minutes

Servings: 8

Ingredients:

- 2 cups rolled oats, pulsed a few times using a food processor

- 1 1/2 cup peanut butter or sunflower butter

- 1/2 cup sunflower seeds

- 1/3 cup honey or maple syrup

- 1/3 cup mini chocolate chips

- 1 teaspoon cinnamon

- 12 teaspoon sea salt, optional

Preparation:

1) Add the oats, peanut butter or sunflower butter, sunflower seeds, honey or maple syrup, and salt, if using, to the bowl of a food processor and combine it together.

2) Add the chocolate chips to the mix and pulse a few more times.

3) Prepare an 8-inch square pan with parchment paper, leaving enough paper to overlap the sides. This will make it easier to get the bars out of the pan when they are done.

4) Transfer the mixture from the food processor to the pan. Using your hands, press it down so that the mixture is really well-pakced.

5) Place the pan in the fridge to set for 30 minutes.

6) Once they are set, take them out by pulling on the ends of the parchment paper, and transferring the bars to a cutting board. Then use a sharp knife or pizza cutter to cut them into bars.

Blueberry and Banana Breakfast Parfaits

Preparation Time: 5 minutes

Cooking Time: 0 minutes

Total Time: 5 minutes

Servings: 1 or more, depending on amount made

Ingredients:

- 1 – 2 bananas, frozen, to taste

- 1 – 2 cups blueberries, frozen, to taste

- 1 – 2 cups dried mulberries, to taste

Preparation:

1) Using a food processor, pulse the dried mulberries until they become crumbles. Transfer to a container and set aside.

2) Next, pulse the bananas while still frozen, creating an "ice cream". Transfer to another container and set aside.

3) Finally, pulse the blueberries while still frozen, creating another "ice cream". Transfer to another container and set aside.

4) In each parfait glass, layer the parfait starting with some of the mulberry crumbles, followed by some of the blueberry "ice cream", followed by some of the banana "ice cream", and repeat until you get to the top of the parfait glass.

Cinnamon Rolls

Preparation Time: 10 minutes

Cooking Time: 0 minutes

Total Time: 10 minutes

Servings: 8

Ingredients:

For the Dough:

- 1 cup almonds or pecan
- 1/2 cup flax seed, ground to a fine powder
- 1/4 cup honey or agave nectar

For the Filling:

- 1/2 cup dates
- 1/4 cup water
- 2 tablespoons cinnamon
- 1 tablespoon coconut oil
- 1/4 teaspoon salt

- 2 tablespoons raisins, optional

- 2 tablespoons pecans or walnuts, chopped, optional

For the "Cream Cheese Icing":

- 1 cup cashews

- 1/4 cup coconut oil

- 4 – 6 tablespoons orange juice or coconut water

- 1 tablespoon honey or agave nectar, optional

- 1 vanilla bean, scraped, optional

Preparation:

For the Dough:

1) Add the almonds or pecans and the ground flax seed to the bowl of a food processor, and blend until you get a flour.

2) Add the honey. Process again until a dough forms, adding a bit of water, if necessary.

3) Transfer the dough to a sheet of wax paper, and add another sheet of wax paper on top.

4) Using a rolling pin, flatten the dough until it's 8- or 9-inch square.

5) Peel off the topmost sheet and set the dough aside.

For the Filling:

1) Add the dates, water, cinnamon, coconut oil, and salt to a blender, and puree it until you get a paste that is thick.

2) Get your dough, and spread the filling evenly over it. Then top with the raisins and nuts if you're using.

3) Carefully roll the dough into a tight roll, much like a sushi roll.

4) Transfer to the fridge to set for 30 minutes.

For the "Cream Cheese Icing":

1) Meanwhile, make the icing by putting all of the icing ingredients together in a high speed blender and then mixing. Add water slowly until you get an icing that is smooth, creamy, and a little bit fluffy.

To Assemble:

1) Once the cinnamon roll is set, slice it into 8 pieces and then top each piece with the icing before serving.

Coconut and Pumpkin Spice Energy Bars

Preparation Time: 20 minutes

Setting Time: 1 hour

Total Time: 1 hour and 20 minutes

Servings: 9

Ingredients:

- 2 cups rolled oats
- 1/2 cup raw walnuts
- 8 dates
- 1/2 cup dried cranberries
- 1/4 cup pumpkin seeds
- 1/4 cup sunflower seeds
- 1/4 cup maple syrup
- 2 tablespoons chia seed powder
- 1 tablespoon lemon juice

- 1 tablespoon coconut oil

- 2 teaspoons pumpkin pie spice

- a dash of salt

- 2 tablespoons dried coconut

- 2 tablespoons dried coconut set aside, for garnish

Preparation:

1) Put some water in a bowl and soak the dates in it for 15 minutes. Then remove the pits.

2) Pulse the walnuts and rolled oats using a food processor until combined.

3) Add the dates. Pulse to combine.

4) Add the rest of the ingredients (except the dried coconut for garnishing). Process until you have a dough forming.

5) Line a 9-inch square baking pan with parchment paper.

6) Transfer the mixture to the baking pan and press it firmly and evenly.

7) Garnish the top of the mixture with the reserved dried coconut.

8) Set in the freezer for at least one hour.

9) Once set, remove the bars from the pan and cut into bars using a sharp knife.

Chapter 3: Main Meal and Side Dish Recipes

Chinese Hot and Sour Cole Slaw

Preparation Time: 20 minutes

Cooking Time: 0 minutes

Total Time: 20 minutes

Servings: 4

Ingredients:

- 3 tablespoons rice vinegar

- 1 tablespoon low sodium soy sauce

- 1 tablespoon toasted sesame oil

- 1 teaspoon fresh ginger, grated
- 1/4 teaspoon white pepper, ground
- 1/4 teaspoon crushed red pepper, to taste
- 3 cups Napa cabbage or green cabbage, shredded
- 1 cup red bell pepper, sliced thinly
- 1/3 cup scallions, sliced
- 8 ounces bamboo shoots, sliced thinly – drained if came from a can

Preparation:

- In a large bowl using a whisk, mix together the soy sauce, oil, ginger, white pepper and crushed red pepper.
- Add the rest of the ingredients. Then give it a toss until it's coated.

Vegan Cream of Mushroom Soup

Preparation Time: 5 minutes

Cooking Time: 5 minutes

Total Time: 10 minutes

Servings: 4 – 6

Ingredients:

- 2 cups cashew milk

- 1/2 of an onion, chopped

- 1 garlic clove

- 1 cup mushrooms plus extra diced mushrooms for garnishing

- 2 tablespoons nama shoyu or liquid aminos

- 1 tablespoon lime juice

- sea salt, to taste

Preparation:

1) Blend all of the ingredients in a blender or food processor until creamy.

2) Garnish with mushrooms before serving.

Ranch Dressing (For Salads, Sandwiches, Etc.)

Preparation Time: 5 minutes

Cooking Time: 0 minutes

Total Time: 5 minutes

Servings: 1

Ingredients:

- 1/2 cup raw cashews, soaked overnight
- 1/2 cup of Persian cucumber, peeled and then chopped.
- 2-inch piece of the white part of a spring onion, chopped
- 1/2 garlic clove, chopped
- 1/4 cup olive oil or avocado oil
- 2 teaspoons apple cider vinegar
- 1/4 teaspoon sea salt
- 3 or more tablespoons of water

- 2 – 3 sprigs of fresh dill, chopped very finely

- 2 – 3 sprigs of fresh basil, chopped very finely

- 10 or more stems fresh chives, to taste, chopped very finely

- 2 – 3 sprigs of fresh Italian parsley, chopped very finely

- 1/4 – 1/2 teaspoon red pepper flakes, optional for a spicier dressing

Preparation:

1) Put the following into the blender: the cashews, cucumber, spring onion, garlic, oil, vinegar, salt, and water (starting with the initial 3 tablespoons).

2) Blend until the dressing is both smooth and creamy. Add more water if you want it thinner. Transfer it to a bowl.

3) Then add the dill, basil, chives, and parsley, and stir it all in. If using, add the red pepper flakes as well.

4) Serve on a salad, as a dip for raw vegetables, or whatever you like.

Carrot Sushi Rolls

Preparation Time: 10 minutes

Cooking Time: 0 minutes

Total Time: 10 minutes

Servings: 2 sushi rolls

Ingredients:

- 2 Nori seaweed sheets
- 4 carrots, peeled and cut
- 1/2 avocado, cut into thick sticks
- 1/2 bell pepper (any color), cut into sticks or julienne-style
- 1/3 kohlrabi, cut into sticks or julienne-style
- low sodium soy sauce, for serving

Preparation:

1) Start with putting the carrots into a food processor and then process until you get a rice-like texture that is also even.

2) Lay out the Nori seaweed sheets onto a work surface.

3) Spread out the carrot "rice" evenly across each of the Nori sheets.

4) Lay out the rest of the vegetables, as well as the avocado, over the carrot layer.

5) Then carefully roll the seaweed up with the vegetables in the center.

6) With a sharp knife, cut the rolls up into 6 to 8 pieces before serving with some low sodium soy sauce.

Spinach Burgers For the Dehydrator

Preparation Time: 10 minutes

Dehydration Time: 8 hours

Total Time: 8 hours and 10 minutes

Servings: 4 – 5

Ingredients:

- 1 cup sunflower seeds

- 3 tablespoons tamari, nama shoyu, or coconut aminos

- 2 cups pulp from green juice, such as from kale, parsley, celery, etc.

- 1/4 cup flax meal

- 2 tablespoons mustard

- 1 tablespoon lemon juice

- 1 teaspoon dried oregano

Preparation:

1) Process the sunflowers in a food processor using an S-blade, until it is well ground.

2) Add the rest of the ingredients and process again until it is well mixed.

3) Line the dehydrator tray with Teflex.

4) Transfer the mixture to a work surface, and then form it into 4 or 5 patties, and place each on the lined dehydrator tray.

5) Dehydrate the patties for 4 hours at 115 degrees. Then flip them over to dehydrate for another 4 hours.

Note: Try serving on the Raw Food Sandwich Bread below!

Raw Food Sandwich Bread

Preparation Time: 10 minutes

Dehydration Time: 6 – 8 hours

Total Time: 6 hours 10 minutes to 8 hours and 10 minutes

Servings: 12 slices

Ingredients:

- 3 cups buckwheat, soaked overnight and then rinsed
- 1 1/2 cups sunflower seeds, soaked for 4 hours and then rinsed
- 1 teaspoon turmeric
- 1/2 teaspoon onion powder
- 1/2 teaspoon garlic powder
- 2 1/2 teaspoon garam masala powder

- 1 1/2 teaspoon Himalayan salt

- 1 tablespoon coconut oil

- 1/3 cup raw coconut water or purified water

- 1 small zucchini

- 1/4 cup yellow onion

Preparation:

1) Add all of the ingredients to a food processor and blend it together until you get a dough.

2) Spread the mixture evenly onto your dehydrator sheets, making sure each piece is about a 1/8 inch thick and spread nearly to the edge of each sheet.

3) Dehydrate for 6 to 8 hours at 110 to 115 degrees.

4) Once done, keep the leftovers in a cool, dry place for up to 5 to 7 days. Alternatively, you can store them in the fridge and then re-dehydrate them for 20 minutes before using.

Veggie Sandwich on Onion Bread

Preparation Time: 10 minutes

Dehydration Time: 3 hours

Total Time: 3 hours and 10 minutes

Servings: 1

Ingredients:

For the Onion Bread:

- 1 cup flax seeds, ground
- 1 cup purified water
- 3 medium onions, sliced thinly
- 2 large carrots, grated
- 1 teaspoon salt
- 3 tablespoons olive oil

For the Cashew Mayonnaise

- 1/2 cup cashew
- 1/2 teaspoon garlic powder
- 1 teaspoon agave

For the Sandwich:

- 2 tomato slices

- 1 – 2 lettuce leaves

- 1 -2 (additional) slices onion

Preparation:

For the Onion Bread:

1) Mix the flax seeds with the water in a bowl, and let sit for several minutes to gel.

2) In a separate bowl, stir together the thinly sliced onion and grated carrots. Then add the salt.

3) Spread the mixture out onto a lined dehydrator sheet. Dehydrate for about an hour or so at 110 degrees.

4) Check to see if the top is a little dry to the touch, flip over, and then dehydrate for another couple of hours, until the bread is dry but not brittle.

For the Cashew Mayonnaise:

1) Put all of the mayo into a high efficiency blender and puree until smooth and creamy.

To Assemble:

1) Lay out the bread slices. On each side, spread out a bit of the cashew mayo. Then lay out the veggies, put together, and serve.

Raw Taco Meat Wraps

Preparation Time: 5 minutes

Cooking Time: 0 minutes

Total Time: 5 minutes

Servings: 4

Ingredients:

- 1 cup walnuts
- 1/3 cup sundried tomatoes, soaked in oil
- 1 1/2 tablespoons olive oil
- 1/2 tablespoon chili powder
- 1/8 teaspoon cayenne pepper
- 1/4 teaspoon sea salt
- 4 lettuce leaves
- raw salsa (see recipe here), optional
- other possible add-ons: avocado, corn, etc.

Preparation:

1) Process all of the ingredients together in a food processor until you get a texture that somewhat looks like taco meat.

2) Divide the meat onto the leaves of lettuce, top with the salsa, if desired, and any other raw toppings desired. Wrap up and enjoy!

Raw Gazpacho

Preparation Time: 5 minutes

Cooking Time: 0 minutes

Total Time: 5 minutes

Note: total time does not include chilling time

Servings: 2

Ingredients:

For the Soup:

- 4 tomatoes, diced
- 1/2 of a medium white onion, diced
- 1 garlic clove, peeled and then minced
- lemon juice, to taste
- 1 cucumber, peeled and then chopped

For Garnish:

- 4 tablespoons fresh cilantro, chopped
- the green part of 1 scallion, chopped finely
- 1 red bell pepper, seeded, cored, and then diced

- 1 tablespoon raw virgin olive oil

- 1/4 cup mango, diced into small cubes

Preparation:

1) Add all of the soup ingredients (leave out the garnish ingredients) to a blender and puree it all together.

2) Strain.

3) Transfer to a bowl and chill overnight.

4) Garnish with the garnish ingredients before serving.

Moroccan Salad

Preparation Time: 15 minutes

Cooking Time: 0 minutes

Total Time: 15 minutes

Note: total time does not include marinating time, if you choose to do so.

Servings: 1 – 2

Ingredients:

- 3 carrots, spiralized into noodles
- 2 tablespoons cilantro, chopped
- the green part of 1 green onion, chopped
- 3 tablespoons orange juice
- 2 teaspoons lemon juice

- 2 teaspoons (raw) extra virgin olive oil

- 1/4 teaspoon cumin, ground

- 1/8 teaspoon sea salt

- a dash of cinnamon

- a dash of cayenne pepper

- a dash of black pepper, freshly ground

Preparation:

1) In a mixing bowl, mix the cilantro and green onion in with the carrot "noodles".

2) Whisk together the orange juice, lemon juice, olive oil, salt, cumin, cinnamon, cayenne pepper, and black pepper in a separate bowl until it is well combined. This will be the dressing.

3) Pour the dressing over the carrot "noodles".

4) Serve immediately or place in the fridge to let marinate for a few hours.

Veggie Pasta Marinara

Preparation Time: 5 minutes

Cooking Time: 0 minutes – see note at the bottom

Total Time: 5 minutes

Servings: 4

Ingredients:

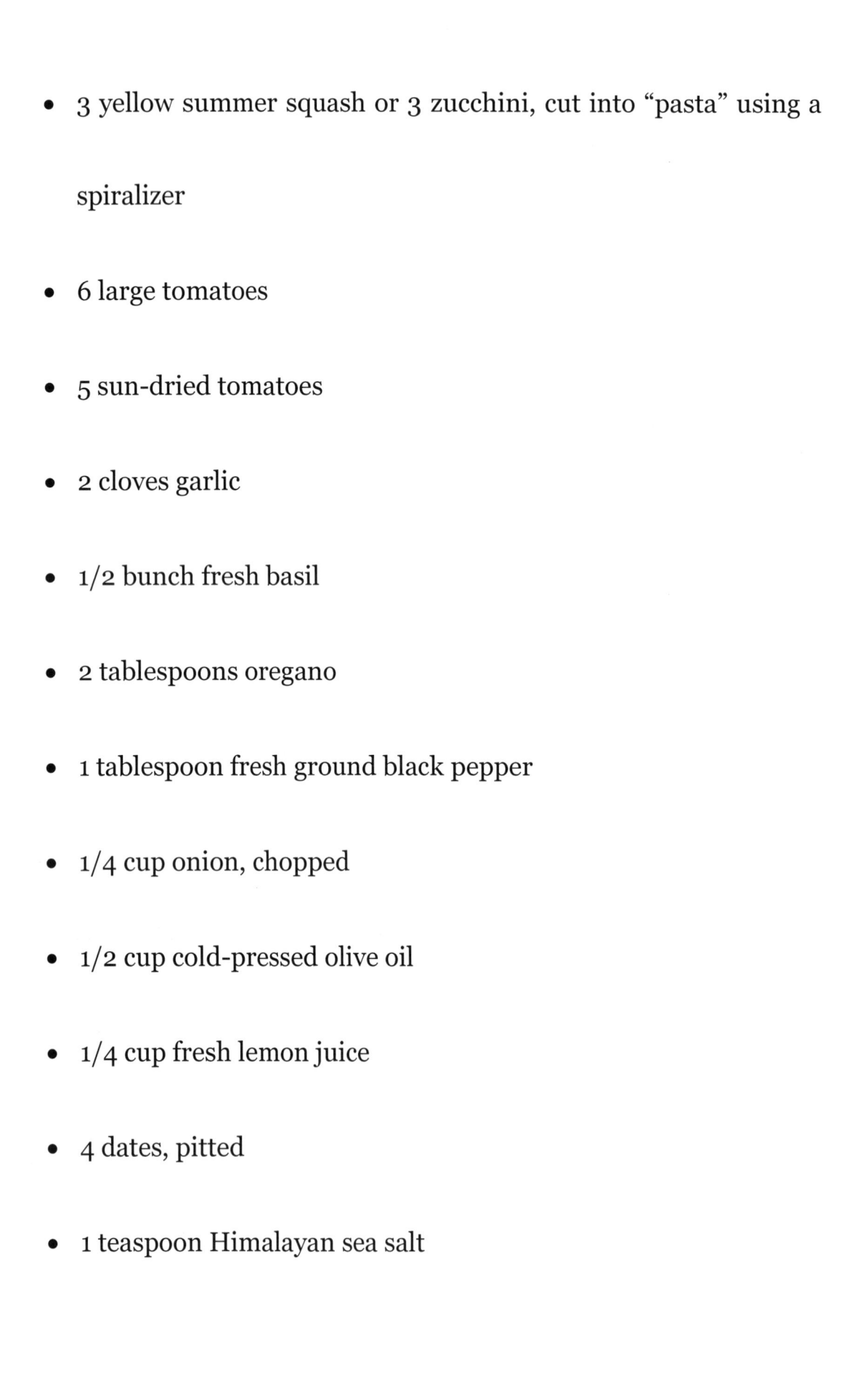

- 3 yellow summer squash or 3 zucchini, cut into "pasta" using a spiralizer
- 6 large tomatoes
- 5 sun-dried tomatoes
- 2 cloves garlic
- 1/2 bunch fresh basil
- 2 tablespoons oregano
- 1 tablespoon fresh ground black pepper
- 1/4 cup onion, chopped
- 1/2 cup cold-pressed olive oil
- 1/4 cup fresh lemon juice
- 4 dates, pitted
- 1 teaspoon Himalayan sea salt

Preparation:

1) Put all of the ingredients except the "pasta" into a high-speed blender.

2) Blend until it is creamy. If desired, add a little bit of purified water at a time if you think the sauce is too thick.

3) If needed, move any excess oil off of your veggie pasta before plating and then pouring the sauce on top.

Note: If you prefer a warmer meal, heat the pasta up to 118 degrees Fahrenheit by rinsing it in warm purified water or place in the oven and heat at 70 degrees Fahrenheit.

Cauliflower Rice Pilaf

Preparation Time: 10 minutes

Cooking Time: 0 minutes

Total Time: 10 minutes

Servings: 4

Ingredients:

- 3 cups cauliflower florets, chopped
- 1/2 of a small red onion, chopped
- 1 small fresh clove garlic, peeled and then chopped finely
- 1/2 of an avocado
- 1/2 tablespoon freshly squeezed lemon juice

- 1 1/2 tablespoon extra virgin olive oil

- 1 plum tomato, diced

- 1/2 sweet bell pepper, chopped (any color)

- 1/2 teaspoon chili powder, to taste

- 1/2 teaspoon paprika

- a pinch of cayenne, optional

- 1/2 fresh cilantro, chopped finely

- sea salt, to taste

- freshly ground pepper, to taste

Preparation:

1) Add the cauliflower, onion and garlic to a food processor. Pulse until the cauliflower is finely chopped and has the consistency of rice.

2) Then, mash the avocado in a bowl and add the lemon juice and olive oil, stirring until it is creamy.

3) Then stir in the cauliflower "rice" mix and give it another stir until the "rice" is coated.

4) Next, add the tomato, bell pepper, chili powder, paprika, cayenne and cilantro. Gently stir it up.

5) Finally, season to taste with the salt and pepper before serving.

Zucchini Noodles With "Bolognese" Sauce

Preparation Time: 10 minutes

Cooking Time: 0 minutes

Total Time: 10 minutes

Servings: 2

Ingredients:

- 3 zucchini or 3 carrots, cut into noodles with a spiralizer
- 3 1/2 ounces sun-dried tomatoes
- 3 1/2 ounces walnut
- juice from 1/2 a lemon
- 1 tablespoon pine nut butter
- salt, to taste
- pepper, to taste
- a pinch of chili flakes, to taste

Preparation:

1) Blend the following ingredients together in a blender: the sun-dried tomatoes, lemon juice, and pine nut butter.

2) Add the salt, pepper, and chili flakes, to taste.

3) Now add the walnuts. Give it a pulse a couple of times, but no more than that, so that you still have bits of walnuts in the sauce.

4) Pour the resulting sauce over the noodles and serve.

"Fish" Sticks With Tartar Sauce

For the "Fish" Sticks:

Preparation Time: 10 minutes

Dehydration Time: 5 – 7 hours

Total Time: 5 hours and 10 minutes to 7 hours and 10 minutes

Servings: 20

For the Tartar Sauce:

Preparation Time: 10 minutes

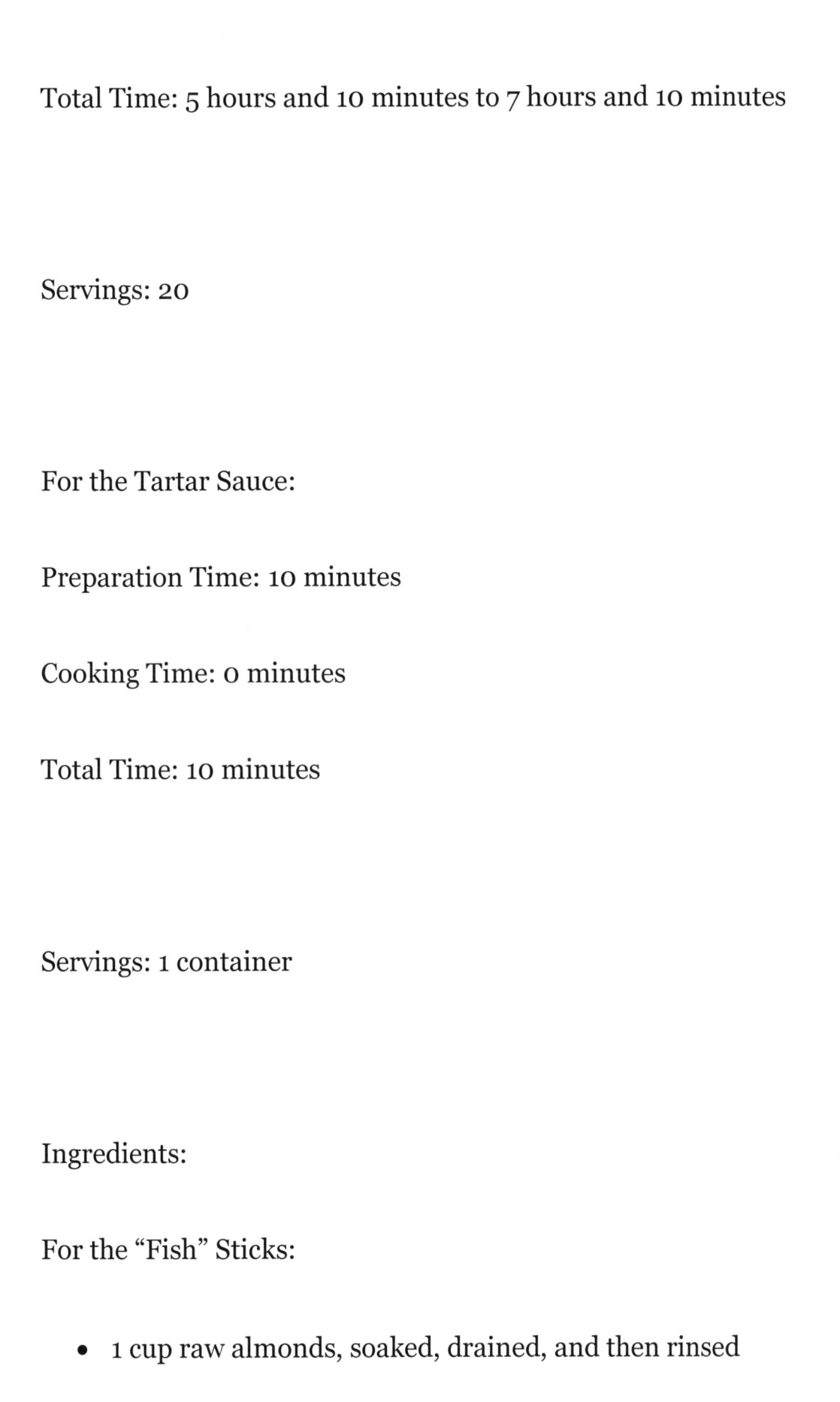

Cooking Time: 0 minutes

Total Time: 10 minutes

Servings: 1 container

Ingredients:

For the "Fish" Sticks:

- 1 cup raw almonds, soaked, drained, and then rinsed

- 1 cup raw sunflower seeds, soaked, drained, and then rinsed
- 1/2 cup celery, minced
- 1/2 cup red onion, minced
- 1/4 cup fresh lime juice
- 1 tablespoon kelp powder plus 1 teaspoon kelp powder, divided
- 1 teaspoon liquid aminos or tamari
- 1 teaspoon sea salt
- 1 tablespoon fresh dill weed
- 1/2 cup water

For the "Breading" For The "Fish" Sticks:

- 1/2 cup raw cashews
- 1/4 cup flax seeds, ground
- 1 teaspoon paprika, smoked

- 1 teaspoon sea salt, smoked

- 1/2 teaspoon black pepper, freshly ground

- 1 teaspoon nutritional yeast

For the Tartar Sauce:

- 1 cup cashews, soaked for 2 hours, drained, and then rinsed

- 1/2 cup water

- 1 tablespoon apple cider vinegar

- 2 teaspoon horseradish powder

- 1 tablespoon pickle juice

- 1/2 teaspoon garlic powder

- 1/2 teaspoon Himalayan pink salt

- 1/2 cup sweet pickle, minced

- 2 tablespoons horseradish, grated, optional

- the white parts of 4 green onions, minced

Preparation:

For the "Fish" Sticks:

1) Add the almonds and sunflower seeds to a food processor with an S-blade. Process until you get a paste.

2) Add the celery, onion, lime juice, kept powder, aminos or tamari, salt, and dill. Blend them together, scraping the sides of the bowl from time to time.

3) With the food processor running, slowly drizzle in the water until you get a nice, moist paste. Transfer it to a bowl.

For the Breading:

1) Using a food processor, grind the cashews into small crumbs without overprocessing.

2) Add the flax seeds, paprika, salt, pepper, and yeast. Pulse it all together and then transfer to a rectangular container big enough to dip the "fish" sticks into.

To Assemble and "Fry":

1) Taking 2 tablespoons of "fish" batter at a time, shape into fish sticks.

2) Dip each "fish" stick into the breading to fully coat both sides.

3) Lay them out on the lined dehydrator tray.

4) Dehydrate starting at 145 degrees for 1 hour. Then reduce heat to 115 and continue for another 4 to 5 hours, until they are moist.

5) Leftovers can be stored in the fridge for up to 5 days and then reheated in the dehydrator.

For the Tartar Sauce:

1) Add the cashews to a blender, followed by the water, vinegar, horseradish powder, pickle juice, garlic powder, and salt. Blend until smooth, about 1 to 5 minutes. Transfer to a bowl.

2) Taste to see if your desired level of horseradish taste is reached. If not, more will be added in the next step.

3) Next add the pickle, onion and, if using, horseradish (a little at a time until desired taste), and then stir it all together.

4) Serve with the "fish" sticks.

5) Leftovers can be stored in an airtight container for up to 5 days.

Raw Pad Thai

Preparation Time: 30 minutes

Cooking Time: 0 minutes

Total Time: 30 minutes

Servings: 4

Ingredients:

- 2 zucchini, ends trimmed and then spiralized into noodles
- 2 carrots, sliced into thin, long sticks
- 1 head red cabbage, sliced thinly
- 1 red bell pepper, sliced thinly
- 1/2 cup bean sprouts
- 3/4 cup raw almond butter
- the juice from 2 oranges
- 2 tablespoons raw honey

- 1 tablespoon fresh ginger root, minced

- 1 tablespoon nama shoyu

- 1 tablespoon unpasteurized miso

- 1 garlic clove, minced

- 1/4 teaspoon cayenne pepper

Preparation:

1) In a large bowl, combine the carrots, cabbage, bell pepper, and bean sprouts.

2) In a separate bowl, using a whisk, mix together the almond butter, orange juice, honey, ginger, nama shoyu, miso, garlic, and cayenne pepper. This will be the sauce.

3) Pour half of the sauce into the cabbage mix and give it a toss until it is coated.

4) Add the sauce-cabbage mix to the zucchini "noodles" and then pour the remainder of the sauce over it.

Vegetable Spring Rolls With Spicy Curry Dipping Sauce

Preparation Time: 20 minutes

Cooking Time: 0 minutes

Total Time: 20 minutes

Servings: 8

Ingredients:

For the Spring Rolls:

- 1 yellow bell pepper, cut into strips

- 3 cups baby spinach

- 1 zucchini, cut julienne-style

- 2 carrots, cut julienne-style

- 3 leaves red cabbage, cut into strips

- 8 rice paper rounds

For the Spicy Curry Dipping Sauce:

- 1/2 cup raw cashews, soaked

- 1 carrot, cubed

- juice from 1 lemon

- 1 teaspoon curry

- 1 teaspoon turmeric

- 1/3 teaspoon cayenne pepper

Preparation:

For the Spring Rolls:

1) Put some warm water in a bowl.

2) Carefully dip each rice paper round into the water for about 5 seconds, until it is soft and flexible to use. Flatten each piece out on your work surface as you go.

3) On the bottom third of each round, lay out some of the spinach.

4) Then top the spinach with some bell pepper, zucchini, carrot, and red cabbage.

5) Fold in the sides of the rice paper, and roll the rice paper up away from you so that it's like a burrito, making sure to tightly tuck in the sides as you go.

6) Once done, place them each on a plate, seam side down.

For the Spicy Curry Dipping Sauce:

1) Put all of the ingredients into a blender or food processor and blend until smooth.

2) Serve with the spring rolls.

Curry Zoodles (Zucchini Noodles)

Preparation Time: 10 minutes

Cooking Time: 0 minutes

Total Time: 10 minutes

Servings: 6

Ingredients:

- 6 ounces coconut water
- 2 cups raw cashews
- 1 large garlic clove
- 1/8 of a large avocado
- 2 teaspoons curry powder
- 1 teaspoon red chili paste
- 1/4 teaspoon cayenne
- 1/4 teaspoon sea salt
- 3 – 4 medium-sized zucchinis, ends chopped and the spiralized into "noodles"

Preparation:

1) Using a high speed blender, blend all of the ingredients, except the zucchini "noodles", together on high until you get a very smooth sauce.

2) Stir the sauce with the zucchini "noodles" until it is completely coated.

Egg-Free Egg Salad

Preparation Time: 10 minutes

Cooking Time: 0 minutes

Total Time: 10 minutes

Servings: 4 – 6

Ingredients:

- 1/2 cup water

- the juice from 1 small lemon

- 1 garlic clove

- 1 teaspoon sea salt, plus more, to taste

- 1 1/2 cups raw cashews

- 1/2 teaspoon dry mustard

- 1/2 teaspoon turmeric, plus more, to taste

- 1 tablespoon apple cider vinegar

Preparation:

1) Using a high speed blender or food processor, blend the water, lemon juice, garlic, sea salt, and cashews until very smooth.

2) Transfer to a medium mixing bowl.

3) Stir in the mustard, apple cider vinegar, and turmeric slowly, taste testing as you go, until you get your desired flavor.

4) Make a sandwich out of it using raw bread or eat on crackers, etc.

Raw Mushroom Burgers With Avocado Mayonnaise

Preparation Time: 25 minutes

Dehydration Time: 4 hours

Total Time: 4 hours and 25 minutes

Servings: 2 or more, depending on size of patties

Ingredients:

For the Burgers:

- 1/2 of a red pepper
- 1/4 cup flax seeds, ground
- 10 ounces mushrooms, cleaned with a soft cloth
- 1/3 cup walnuts
- 1/2 white onion, chopped
- 1 jalapeno pepper, chopped
- 1 rib celery, chopped
- 2 tablespoons olive oil

For the Avocado Mayonnaise:

- 1 ripe avocado

- 1 teaspoon agave nectar
- 1/4 teaspoon salt
- 1/2 teaspoon garlic powder
- 1/2 teaspoon onion powder
- 1 teaspoon paprika
- 1 teaspoon vinegar

Additional Topping Ideas:

- lettuce leaves
- red onion, chopped
- jalapenos, chopped

Preparation:

For the Burger:

1) Use a blender to puree the red pepper until it is liquefied, adding water as needed along the way.

2) Transfer it to a bowl and stir it together with the ground flax seeds. Then let this soak for 15 minutes, until gooey.

3) Fit a food processor with an S blade and the pulse together the mushrooms, walnuts, jalapeno, onion, and celery until it is all finely chopped.

4) Then stir in the flax seed – red pepper mix, plus two tablespoons of olive oil.

5) Take the mixture and form patties, laying them out on a teflex-lined dehydrator tray as you go.

6) Add a little more olive oil to the tray.

7) Dehydrate for 2 hours. Then flip them over, and dehydrate for another 2 hours.

For the Avocado Mayonnaise:

1) Put the ingredients into a blender and then blend until it is creamy.

2) Put it all together on a bed of lettuce leaves, raw sandwich bread or burger buns, etc.

Raw Caesar Salad

Preparation Time: 10 minutes

Cooking Time: 0 minutes

Total Time: 10 minutes

Servings: 1

Ingredients:

- 1/4 cup raw cashews or raw sunflower seeds
- 1/8 cup raw sesame seeds or raw pine nuts or 2 tablespoons tahini
- 1/8 – 1/4 cup sunflower seeds, to desired thickness
- 3 – 4 tablespoons lemon juice, freshly squeezed, to taste
- 1 – 2 medium garlic cloves, chopped, to taste
- 1 1/2 teaspoon mild miso
- 1/2 teaspoon dried dill
- 1 - 2 dates or 1 – 2 teaspoon agave nectar or other liquid sweetener, to taste
- 1/2 – 2/3 cup filtered water, if desired, to making dressing thinner

- black pepper, freshly ground, to taste

Preparation:

1) Combine all of the ingredients and then puree using a blender, until very smooth.

2) Taste. If desired, add additional garlic, lemon juice, and dates or agave nectar.

3) Also check for thickness of the dressing. If desired, add water to thin it out.

Chapter 5: Snack and Dessert Recipes

Fresh and Easy Guacamole

Preparation Time: 10 minutes

Cooking Time: 0 minutes

Total Time: 10 minutes

Servings: 6 – 8

Ingredients:

- 1/2 cup cilantro leaves, coarsely chopped

- 1 jalapeno pepper, finely minced - optional for heat

- 2 cloves garlic, pressed or minced

- 1/2 cup small red onion, diced

- juice from 1 fresh lime (2 tablespoons of bottled lime juice is okay)

- 4 medium Roma tomatoes, diced

- 4 avocados, diced

Preparation:

1) Combine the cilantro leaves, jalapeno, garlic, onion and juice.

2) Add the tomatoes and mix again.

3) Fold in the avocado, gently.

Note: try serving these with the <u>corn tortilla chips</u> from the recipe in this book!

Crunchy Coconut Macaroons

Preparation Time: 10 minutes

Dehydration Time: 12 – 24 hours

Total Time: 12 hours 10 minutes – 24 hours 10 minutes

Servings: 30 – 45 cookies

Ingredients:

- 2 cups almonds, soaked for 8 hours
- 1 cup shredded coconut
- 1 tablespoon almond extract
- 6 – 10 dates, pitted, soaked for 2 hours

Preparation:

1) Put a 1/2 cup of water from the dates, the dates, the almond extract, and the coconut – keeping it double thick – into a blender and blend it up into a dough.

2) Drop balls of the dough on a sheet of wax paper covering the trays of the dehydrator.

3) Dehydrate the cookies at 105 degrees for about 12 to 24 hours, making sure to turn over the dough when it is firm. Cookies will be done when they have reached your desired chewy consistency.

<u>No Bake Strawberry "Cheesecake"</u>

Preparation Time: 20 minutes

Cooking Time: 0 minutes

Total Time: 20 minutes

Note: This does not include time to set the cheesecake in the fridge

Ingredients:

For the Crust:

- 1 1/2 cups raw almonds
- 2/3 cup raisins
- 1/4 cup shredded coconut
- 2 tablespoons filtered water

For the "Cheesecake"

- 3 cups raw cashews

- 3/4 cup lemon juice

- lemon zest from 1 lemon

- 1/2 cup maple syrup or agave nectar

- a pinch of salt

- 1/2 cup coconut oil, melted and then cooled

- 1 pink organic strawberries, reserving 5 or 6 strawberries for decorating the top

Preparation:

1) Place some warm water in a bowl and soak the cashews in it for about 15 minutes. Meanwhile, start making the crust as follows.

For the Crust:

Servings: 16

Ingredients:

- 1 cup rolled oats
- 1/4 cup ground sunflower seeds
- 1/2 cup carob powder
- 1/2 cup honey
- 1/4 cup sesame seeds, toasted and then ground up
- 2 cups walnuts, chopped

Preparation:

1) In a mixing bowl, combine all of the ingredients well.

2) Press the mixture into the bottom of an 8-inch square baking pan or dish.

3) Put in the fridge to chill.

4) Cut into 2-inch squares before serving, using a sharp knife. If they seem a bit crumbly, that's normal.

Raw Salsa With Raw Corn Tortilla Chips

For the Salsa:

Preparation Time: 10 minutes

Cooking Time: 0 minutes

Total Time: 10 minutes

Servings: 2 cups

For the Corn Tortilla Chips:

Preparation Time: 5 minutes

Dehydration Time: 15 – 17 hours

Total Time: 15 hours 5 minutes to 17 hours 5 minutes

Servings: 4 or more, depending on size of chips after cutting

Ingredients:

For the Salsa

- 2 cups tomatoes, chopped into small pieces
- 1 – 2 garlic cloves, pressed or minced
- 1/4 teaspoon sea salt, to taste
- juice from 1/2 a lime
- optional:

2 tablespoons fresh cilantro, minced

1 tablespoon red onion, minced

1/2 teaspoon cumin, ground

1/2 teaspoon chili powder

1/4 teaspoon cayenne powder

1 teaspoon chili pepper of choice, minced

For the Corn Tortilla Chips:

- 4 corn on the cob, kernels shaved off, reserving a 1/2 cup
- juice from 2 limes
- 1/4 cup of olive oil
- 1 cup sunflower seeds
- 1/2 red bell pepper
- 2 tablespoons coriander
- 2 tablespoons dried basil

- 1 garlic clove, chopped

- 1 tablespoon of miso paste

Preparation:

For the Salsa:

1) Combine all of the ingredients, including any optional ingredients into a large bowl and mix it gently to combine.

2) Chill in the fridge while you make the chips.

For the Corn Tortilla Chips:

1) Use a high speed blender to blend all of the ingredients except the reserved 1/2 cup of kernels.

2) Transfer to a mixing bowl and then add the 1/2 cup of reserved kernels back. Mix thoroughly.

3) Transfer the final mixture to a Teflex-lined dehydrator tray.

4) Dehydrate at 105 degrees for 12 to 14 hours, until the chips are firm. After the first hour, use a knife to score out chip-shaped pieces, leaving the mixture in to dehydrate the rest of the way.

5) Once done dehydrating, carefully remove the tray and flip the chips over onto a mesh sheet. Then peel off the Teflex liner.

6) Dehydrate for another few hours until the chips are nice and chip-like.

Note: These chips also go great with the guacamole recipe above.

Raw Oatmeal Raisin Cookies

Preparation Time: 10 minutes

Dehydration Time: 12 hours

Total Time: 12 hours and 10 minutes

Servings: 12

Ingredients:

- 2 cups oat groats
- 1/2 cup almonds
- 1/2 cup raisins
- 1/2 cup agave nectar or maple syrup
- 1/4 cup cashews

Preparation:

1) Grind the oat groats until fine, using a food processor. Transfer to a bowl.

2) Next, put the almonds into the food processor and only pulse them a few times, enough for them to just about be coarsely chopped. Transfer to the bowl with the oat groats.

3) Now add the raisins and sweetener of choice (agave or maple syrup) to the oat – almond mix. Mix well.

4) Use a coffee grinder to grind the cashews and then coat your hands in them like flour in order to handle the cookie batter.

5) In small chunks, roll the batter into balls and place them on a mesh sheet-lined dehydrator tray.

6) Dehydrate at 110 degrees for 12 hours, checking to see if you have reached your desired chewiness or crunchiness.

Raw Pumpkin Pie

Preparation Time: 25 minutes

Chilling Time: 30 minutes

Total Time: 55 minutes

Servings: 1 pie

Ingredients:

For the Crust:

- 2 cups macadamia, almond, or other nut of choice

- 1 1/2 cups medjool dates or other soft date of choice

For the Filling:

- 4 cups pumpkin cubes, skin and seeds removed
- 1 1/2 cups banana, sliced
- 3/4 cup agave nectar
- 1 teaspoon cinnamon
- 1/4 teaspoon nutmeg
- 1 tablespoon lemon juice
- 1/2 teaspoon coriander, ground, optional
- 1/4 teaspoon allspice, optional
- a pinch cayenne, optional

Preparation:

For the Crust:

1) Using a food processor fitted with an S-blade, grind the nut of choice.

2) Then add the dates, and process for another 40 seconds, until you have a sticky mixture that sticks to the sides of the bowl without the center falling in. If needed you can add more agave nectar to accomplish this, 1 teaspoon at a time. The result needs to be sticky enough to hold together when pressed with your fingers.

3) Transfer the mixture to a pie plate and then press it down and across into a pie crust.

For the Filling:

1) Add all of the ingredients to a high powered blender. Blend on high speed until you get a puree-like texture.

2) Transfer the filling into your pie crust and put in the fridge to chill for at least 30 minutes.

Strawberry Ice Cream

Preparation Time: 10 minutes

Freezing Time = ice cream maker + freezer: 2 hours and 20 minutes,

or more, depending on your ice cream maker

Total Time: 2 hours and 30 minutes, or more

Servings: 1 container

Ingredients:

- 2 cups fresh strawberries, hulled and then cut into quarters

- 1/2 cup almond milk or hemp milk

- 1 cup coconut milk

- 1/2 cup turbinado sugar

- 1/2 teaspoon vanilla extract (alcohol-free, if desired)

- a tiny pinch of salt

Preparation:

1) Using a high powered blender, blend together the strawberries, almond or hemp milk, coconut milk, sugar, vanilla, and salt, until smooth.

2) Transfer it to an ice cream maker and freeze according to instructions for your maker.

3) Transfer to a storage container that is freezer-proof and has a lid. Then place in your freezer to chill for at least 2 hours.

Dark Chocolate Milkshake

Preparation Time: 5 minutes

Cooking Time: 0 minutes

Total Time: 5 minutes

Servings: 1

Ingredients:

- 1 cup almond milk

- 1 teaspoon vanilla extract

- 2 avocados

- 1/2 scant cup agave nectar or other sweetener of choice, plus more if desired

- 1/2 cup raw cacao powder

- a dash of salt

- a dash of cinnamon

- 1 cup ice

Preparation:

1) Put everything, except the ice, into a blender until it is smooth and thick.

2) Add some of the ice, and blend again.

3) Check for sweetness. If you want it sweeter, add more sweetener.

Note: For a thinner milkshake, add additional almond milk, a little at a time, until desired thinness.

Bean-Free Hummus

Preparation Time: 10 minutes

Cooking Time: 0 minutes

Total Time: 10 minutes

Servings: 1 bowl

Ingredients:

- 2 cups zucchini, peeled and chopped

- 1/2 cup sesame seeds, hulled

- the juice from 1 lemon

- 1 teaspoon paprika

- 1/4 teaspoon sea salt, optional

Preparation:

1) Using a food processor, pulse the sesame seeds until they are ground up.

2) Then add the rest of the ingredients, and blend until it is smooth and creamy.

I hope this book will inspire you and you will strive your level best to

avoid obesity and to stay healthy. Stay happy, stay fit.

1) Using a food processor, process the almonds until you get a fine texture.

2) Then add the raisins and coconut. Process, adding a tablespoon of water at a time, until you get a texture that is sticky.

3) Transfer and press into the bottom of a spring form cake pan.

For the "Cheesecake":

1) Now drain the cashews well. Add them to the food processor and pulse until they are ground finely.

2) Then add the lemon juice, lemon zest, agave or maple syrup, and the salt. Mix until it is well blended.

3) Next, add the cooled coconut oil and process it some more.

4) Finally, add the strawberries, except for the reserved ones for decorating, and mix one more time.

5) Pour the "cheesecake" mixture into the crust and put in the fridge until it is set.

6) Once set, decorate the top with the reserved strawberries. Use a sharp knife to slice it into slices.

No Bake Brownies

Preparation Time: 5 minutes

Cooking Time: 0 minutes

Total Time: 5 minutes

Note: This does not include chilling time.